Arachnoiditis Diet Plan

Anti-Inflammatory Meals, Flare-Reduction Strategies & Simple Recipes for Nerve Pain Support

mf

Disclaimer

This guide is provided for informational and educational purposes only and should not be interpreted as medical, nutritional, or professional advice. The author is not a licensed physician, nurse, dietitian, or mental health provider. Reading this guide does not establish a patient–provider relationship of any kind.

Always seek the guidance of a qualified healthcare professional before starting, changing, or discontinuing any supplement, diet, or lifestyle program. If you are pregnant, breastfeeding, managing a chronic medical condition, or taking prescription medications, consult your physician or pharmacist before considering any product mentioned in this guide.

The author and publisher make no representations or warranties regarding accuracy, applicability, fitness, or completeness of the information contained herein. While every effort has been made to ensure scientific accuracy and currency, medical knowledge and research evolve continually. Readers are responsible for verifying information and making decisions in consultation with licensed professionals.

Use of this guide and any information contained within it is at your own risk. The author and publisher disclaim all liability for any loss, injury, or adverse outcome that may result from the use or misuse of this material.

No supplement, diet, or practice discussed in this text is intended to diagnose, treat, cure, or prevent any disease. No outcomes or benefits are guaranteed.

Product names, supplement formulations, diet frameworks, and trademarks mentioned are the property of their respective owners and are used for identification only. Any images or illustrations that appear in related materials are licensed stock or educational placeholders.

Table of Contents

Introduction

Arachnoiditis is a complex neurological condition characterized by inflammation of the arachnoid mater, the delicate membrane that surrounds the brain and spinal cord. This inflammation can result from causes such as trauma, infections, or complications following spinal procedures, and leads to a range of symptoms that can be both chronic and deeply disruptive.

The most prominent among these is persistent nerve pain, often described as burning, stinging, or electric shock-like, which significantly impacts quality of life for those affected. The pain is largely a result of both direct nerve irritation and ongoing inflammatory processes within the central nervous system, making everyday activities challenging and sometimes overwhelming for patients with arachnoiditis.

Chronic nerve pain and inflammation are tightly interwoven in arachnoiditis. As inflammation persists, the nerve tissue is damaged further, causing neuropathic symptoms to intensify and often spread. This cycle can lead to heightened sensitivity in the nervous system, resulting in symptoms such as muscle cramps, numbness, tingling, and even mobility issues.

Managing this inflammatory cascade is therefore a central goal in reducing the frequency and severity of nerve pain associated with the condition. While medications and interventional therapies play a vital role, research increasingly supports the power of nutrition as a foundational and complementary strategy.

Diet can have a direct influence on the body's inflammatory processes, with certain foods and dietary patterns shown to exacerbate or reduce inflammation at the cellular level. Diets high in processed sugars, saturated fats, and artificial additives are linked to increased inflammatory markers, whereas nutrient-rich, whole food diets have been associated with lower levels of systemic inflammation and improved pain outcomes in chronic conditions. Nutritional modulation not only targets the inflammatory response but may also help regulate oxidative stress and support nerve cell repair, offering a valuable adjunct to medical management for individuals with arachnoiditis.

The primary objective of adopting an anti-inflammatory diet plan for arachnoiditis is to calm ongoing inflammation, stabilize nerve function, and support overall well-being. By emphasizing foods that are rich in omega-3 fatty acids, antioxidants, and phytonutrients, and by limiting ingredients that promote inflammation, it is possible to create a dietary environment more conducive to nerve healing and pain control.

The goals include improving day-to-day comfort, lowering the risk of flare-ups, and augmenting the effectiveness of other therapies. Additionally, proper nutrition can help patients maintain a healthy weight, reduce fatigue, and optimize digestion—all factors relevant to those managing chronic pain syndromes.

In this guide, you will discover:

- Step-by-step support for making dietary changes that can make a real difference
- Proven strategies for meal planning, food selection, and preparation
- Practical tools for identifying personal dietary triggers and managing setbacks
- Evidence-based recommendations on what to eat and what to limit
- A collection of simple, flavorful recipes tailored for nerve pain support
- Guidance on supplementation, mindful eating, and strategies for long-term sustainability

If you are newly diagnosed or have been managing arachnoiditis for years, this guide equips you to use nutrition as a powerful ally in reducing inflammation and nerve pain. With focused information and actionable insights, you'll be able to move toward symptom relief and improved quality of life, one meal at a time.

Understanding Arachnoiditis and Its Impact

To understand the profound impact of arachnoiditis, it is essential first to become familiar with the anatomical structures it affects, the pathways through which it develops, and how its symptoms evolve to alter daily life. This chapter explores the core concepts behind the condition, guiding readers through the role of the arachnoid mater within the central nervous system, how arachnoiditis commonly arises, its principal symptoms, possible complications, and the biological underpinnings that drive its relentless progression.

Description of the Arachnoid Mater and Central Nervous System

At the heart of arachnoiditis is the arachnoid mater, a thin, web-like membrane and one of the three primary meninges that envelop the brain and spinal cord. These three layers, known as the dura mater (the tough outer layer), the arachnoid mater (the delicate middle layer), and the pia mater (the innermost membrane), work together to protect the central nervous system (CNS) from injury and infection.

The arachnoid mater specifically occupies a crucial role, acting as a cushioning structure sandwiched between the hard dura mater and the softer pia mater. Beneath the arachnoid lies the cerebrospinal fluid (CSF), a clear, nourishing fluid that both bathes the CNS and acts as a shock absorber.

The central nervous system itself is the command center for body function, made up of the brain and the spinal cord. These structures coordinate everything from movement and sensation to memory and emotion. Consequently, any process that disturbs the meninges, and thus the flow of CSF or the function of neural pathways, can have far-reaching effects. The fragility of the arachnoid mater, combined with its proximity to sensitive neural tissue, makes it particularly vulnerable to damage. ***When it becomes inflamed, as occurs in arachnoiditis***, this sets off a cascade of disruptions throughout the nervous system, often leading to persistent pain and loss of neurological function.

Common Causes of Arachnoiditis

Arachnoiditis is not a disease that arises spontaneously, it is triggered by distinct underlying events or exposures. The three most common causes, each with specific risk factors, are physical trauma, infectious processes, and medical or surgical interventions involving the spine.

1. **Trauma:**

   Direct mechanical injury to the spine, such as might occur with a vertebral fracture, spinal cord injury, or even repeated minor insults, can compromise the integrity of the arachnoid mater. In many cases, this trauma produces bleeding, scarring, or the introduction of debris into the subarachnoid space, providing a trigger for inflammation.

2. **Infection:**

   Infections affecting the central nervous system can reach the meninges, causing inflammatory conditions known as meningitis. When bacterial, viral, or fungal agents specifically attack the arachnoid layer, they can lead to intense inflammatory responses. Even after the infection resolves, lingering scar tissue and adhesions may remain, perpetuating the symptoms of arachnoiditis.

3. **Spinal Procedures:**

   Unfortunately, many cases of arachnoiditis are iatrogenic, meaning they are induced by medical or surgical procedures. Lumbar punctures (spinal taps), epidural injections, and spinal surgeries are all potential triggers. Repeated procedures, the use of certain contrast dyes, and the introduction of foreign materials (like silicone-based compounds) are known to increase the risk. Even the simple act of disturbing spinal tissues can, in susceptible individuals, set off a persistent and unrelenting inflammatory response.

A smaller proportion of cases arises from less common sources, such as exposure to harmful chemicals that inadvertently reach the spinal canal or from chronic degenerative conditions that erode spinal structures over time.

Key Symptoms Including Neuropathic Pain and Sensory Changes

The hallmark of arachnoiditis is chronic, often severe pain with neuropathic qualities. However, this is often accompanied by a constellation of additional symptoms, many of which relate to the disruption of normal nerve signaling.

- ***Neuropathic Pain***: This type of pain is usually described as burning, stinging, stabbing, or electric shock-like. Unlike typical musculoskeletal aches, neuropathic pain in arachnoiditis often defies standard pain relief. It can be relentless, deep-seated, and sometimes migratory, varying in intensity from day to day.
- ***Sensory Changes***: Alongside pain, patients may notice numbness, tingling, or a sensation of insects crawling on the skin. These feelings might be localized or may spread depending on how many nerve roots are

affected. Some people experience marked hypersensitivity, where even gentle touch or clothing contact triggers exaggerated pain responses (allodynia).

- ***Motor Impairment***: As the condition progresses, weakness in the legs may develop, ranging from mild fatigue to profound difficulty with walking or even paralysis in severe cases.
- ***Autonomic Dysfunction***: Because the spinal cord regulates many involuntary functions, people with arachnoiditis can face problems with bowel, bladder, and sexual function. This can include urinary urgency or retention, constipation, or problems with sexual arousal and function. In some cases, sweating and skin temperature regulation are also affected.

Symptoms often fluctuate, with periods of intensification ("flares") followed by partial remission. The unpredictability contributes to emotional distress and affects a person's ability to maintain routines.

Long-term Complications Affecting Mobility and Quality of Life

Living with arachnoiditis extends far beyond physical pain, the condition exerts a profound impact on daily activities, independence, and emotional well-being.

Mobility is particularly susceptible to decline. Chronic nerve inflammation and resultant scarring (known as adhesions) can bind nerve roots together or to surrounding tissues, drastically impeding the transmission of impulses that govern movement. Over time, this may result in gait disturbances, muscle wasting, and an increased risk of falls. Some patients require canes, walkers, or wheelchairs for daily mobility as the disorder progresses.

Quality of life is affected not only by physical limitations but also by sleep disturbances from pain, loss of employment or reduced ability to work, and diminished participation in social activities. Fatigue, depression, and anxiety are common companions, stemming both from the chronic pain itself and from the sense of unpredictability and loss of control that the disease brings.

Additionally, long-term complications may include:

- Progressive neurological decline due to recurrent nerve damage.
- Chronic infections or skin breakdown from reduced mobility.
- Secondary orthopedic problems, such as joint stiffness and pressure sores.

These impacts can form a cycle, in which pain limits movement, reduced movement leads to additional impairment, and emotional distress exacerbates physical symptoms.

Role of Inflammation and Nerve Dysfunction in Symptom Manifestation

Arachnoiditis is an inflammatory disorder of the central nervous system. When the arachnoid mater is disturbed, the body responds by sending immune cells to the site of injury or infection. This inflammatory cascade releases a mix of cytokines and other chemicals designed to contain damage, but in doing so, these agents also sensitize and irritate nerve roots. Instead of aiding healing, chronic inflammation ultimately damages nerve cells and the fibers that conduct signals along the spinal cord.

This ongoing immune response transforms the character of the tissue: the arachnoid thickens, nerve roots may become embedded in fibrous scar tissue, and interconnections—called adhesions—may bind them together abnormally. The altered anatomy leads to persistent pain and disturbed function.

Critically, nerve dysfunction does not simply mean loss of feeling or control. Nerve fibers may begin to fire haphazardly, sending false pain signals or creating sensations in the absence of true stimulation. Damaged nerves can also lose their capacity to regulate bowel and bladder properly or to coordinate muscle activity, compounding the effect. Furthermore, because the pain persists, it can cause what is known as central sensitization, where the CNS becomes increasingly responsive to even minor stimuli, making pain management gradually more challenging.

Understanding how arachnoiditis arises and manifests is the first step toward managing its impact. Those affected should work with healthcare professionals familiar with the condition and track their symptoms carefully to identify triggers for flares. Being informed about the role of inflammation and nerve dysfunction helps guide decisions not only about medical treatment but also about daily lifestyle adaptations, including diet, activity, and stress management.

While much of arachnoiditis is beyond an individual's immediate control, recognizing the ways in which chronic inflammation drives symptoms provides hope. By addressing inflammation through medical, nutritional, and lifestyle strategies, many people with arachnoiditis can take meaningful steps to improve comfort, preserve mobility, and regain a measure of quality in daily life.

Inflammation and Nerve Pain: Dietary Connections

For anyone living with arachnoiditis, chronic pain is more than a symptom, it is a constant presence that can define daily experience. Central to this persistent pain is inflammation, a complex process that can both serve to protect and, under chronic conditions, drive nerve damage and amplify discomfort.

Understanding the relationship between inflammation, nerve pain, and dietary choices is fundamental for anyone seeking to manage their symptoms and improve their quality of life. This chapter explores critical connections, translating emerging research into practical guidance designed to empower meaningful dietary change for nerve pain support.

Chronic Inflammation as a Driver of Neuropathic Pain

Chronic inflammation stands out as a key factor in the development and persistence of neuropathic pain, the type most often reported by those with arachnoiditis. Unlike acute inflammation, which helps heal injury or infection, chronic inflammation can linger, continually activating the immune system in ways that harm rather than heal.

This ongoing response affects nerve fibers, both at the site of spinal injury and throughout the central nervous system, leading to increased sensitivity and spontaneous pain signals even in the absence of obvious triggers. Studies indicate that continued inflammatory activity can promote the release of cytokines and other signaling molecules that sensitize nerves, ultimately amplifying pain transmission and creating feedback loops that sustain discomfort.

The relationship between nerve inflammation and pain is dynamic. Nerves exposed to inflammatory mediators become more excitable and less able to filter out normal stimuli. This not only exacerbates daily pain but can also lead to unusually severe responses from minor aggravations. For people with arachnoiditis, managing inflammation may be one of the most powerful tools in reducing overall pain intensity, frequency, and the unpredictable nature of flares.

Pro-Inflammatory vs. Anti-Inflammatory Foods

Not all foods have the same effect on the body's inflammatory processes. Decades of nutritional science have revealed clear dietary patterns that either promote or help resolve chronic inflammation. Pro-inflammatory foods often contain refined carbohydrates, excessive added sugars, saturated and trans fats, and processed ingredients. These foods—found in sugary soft drinks, white bread, pastries, processed snacks, and fried items may encourage inflammatory pathways at the cellular level, increasing production of cytokines that perpetuate nerve irritation and pain.

Conversely, anti-inflammatory foods provide nutrients and bioactives that can help dampen inflammatory signals. These include:

- ***Fatty fish are rich in omega-3 fatty acids (such as salmon, sardines, and mackerel)***, which can reduce the synthesis of pro-inflammatory molecules and support nerve membrane stability.
- ***Colorful fruits and vegetables, especially berries, kale, spinach, and broccoli***, are known for their high content of flavonoids and antioxidants that neutralize inflammation-inducing free radicals.
- ***Nuts, seeds, and plant oils (like olive oil and flaxseed)*** that provide healthy fats and micronutrients believed to shift immune activity away from chronic inflammation.
- ***Herbs and spices, such as turmeric, ginger, and garlic,*** which contain natural compounds with evidence for anti-inflammatory action in nerve pain models.

The dietary pattern most consistently linked to reduced inflammation and nerve pain is one that prioritizes whole, minimally processed plants; high-quality proteins; and a diverse range of herbs and spices. Such a pattern, much like the Mediterranean diet has been associated with improvements in pain scores and markers of systemic inflammation.

Impact of Blood Sugar Regulation on Nerve Sensitivity

Diet influences more than just inflammation; it also plays a critical role in managing blood sugar levels, which are directly linked to nerve health and pain perception. Spikes and rapid fluctuations in blood glucose can worsen already-sensitized nerves, increasing the risk of neuropathic symptoms such as burning, tingling, and shooting pains.In people with metabolic vulnerabilities or diabetes, poor blood sugar control is a major risk factor for the development and progression of neuropathic pain.

Even for individuals without metabolic disorders, high-glycemic foods; such as sugary cereals, white rice, and processed snacks can provoke glycemic swings that heighten nerve reactivity and inflammation. In contrast, choosing foods with a lower glycemic index (such as legumes, whole grains, and most vegetables) helps maintain steady energy levels and may buffer nerves from damaging inflammatory surges.

Practical strategies for stabilizing blood sugar and supporting nerve health include:

- Combining carbohydrate-containing foods with sources of protein and healthy fat to slow digestion and reduce glucose spikes.
- Prioritizing fiber-rich grains, lentils, beans, and vegetables over processed and refined starches.
- Spacing meals consistently throughout the day to avoid both excessive hunger and erratic overeating.

Gut Microbiome Influence on Systemic Inflammation

Increasingly, science points toward a vital role for the gut microbiome in governing systemic inflammation and, by extension, nerve pain. The human digestive tract is home to trillions of microbes that interact with our immune system, signaling molecules that regulate inflammation and even the metabolism of neurotransmitters implicated in pain pathways. An imbalance in the intestinal flora (dysbiosis), often fueled by processed food or antibiotic use, can promote leaky gut and increased absorption of inflammatory substances into the bloodstream.

Research links diets high in fiber, plant diversity, and fermented foods (such as yogurt with live cultures, kefir, and sauerkraut) with increased populations of beneficial bacteria and reduced markers of inflammation.These dietary elements help maintain the integrity of the intestinal barrier, regulate immune responses, and may reduce pain sensitivity by modulating inflammatory messengers throughout the body.

For those managing chronic nerve pain, supporting gut health can take several practical forms:

- Including a variety of fiber-rich fruits, vegetables, whole grains, and legumes every day to feed beneficial bacteria.
- Incorporating moderate amounts of fermented foods for probiotic support where tolerated.
- Limiting excessive antibiotics unless medically necessary, as these can disrupt healthy microbial populations.

Oxidative Stress and Its Link to Dietary Antioxidants

Oxidative stress occurs when an imbalance between harmful free radicals (reactive oxygen species) and the body's antioxidant defenses causes cellular damage, including damage to sensitive nerve cells. Chronic pain states, including those in arachnoiditis are often characterized by increased oxidative stress, which can further inflame nerves and reinforce pain signaling.

Diet plays a pivotal role in both the production of and defense against oxidative stress. Diets lacking in colorful produce, polyphenols, and certain vitamins tend to be low in the antioxidants needed to neutralize free radicals, while processed foods and unhealthy fats can accelerate their formation. Antioxidant-rich diets which are naturally high in berries, dark leafy greens, nuts, seeds, and a variety of vibrant vegetables help counteract oxidative injury and can help dampen the pain-perpetuating cycle of neuroinflammation.

Key dietary antioxidants for nerve health include:

- ***Vitamin C (abundant in citrus fruits, bell peppers, and strawberries)***, which supports collagen production and immune function while scavenging free radicals.
- ***Vitamin E (found in nuts, seeds, and avocados)***, an essential lipid-soluble antioxidant that helps protect nerve cell membranes.
- ***Polyphenols and flavonoids (present in berries, grapes, green tea, and cocoa)***, which have demonstrated anti-inflammatory and neuroprotective effects in experimental studies.

In practical terms, aiming for a "rainbow" of produce daily is a reliable strategy to naturally boost antioxidant intake. Meals built with a variety of fruits, vegetables, nuts, and seeds not only provide protection against oxidative stress but also contribute valuable nutrients that promote overall nerve healing and resilience.

Identifying and managing drivers of chronic inflammation can offer substantial pain relief and resilience for individuals with arachnoiditis and similar nerve pain conditions. Science consistently highlights an anti-inflammatory dietary pattern rich in whole, plant-based foods, healthy fats, proteins, and abundant antioxidants as a supportive foundation for nerve health. At the same time, minimizing pro-inflammatory foods, stabilizing blood sugar, nurturing the gut microbiome, and filling the plate with antioxidants are not isolated actions; they work synergistically to calm the body's responses and offer the best chance for sustained improvement in nerve-related symptoms.

With this knowledge, you can begin to make purposeful adjustments in your food choices and eating habits. The following chapters will guide you through selecting supportive foods, preparing simple, anti-inflammatory meals, and integrating these insights into a lifelong approach to better nerve health.

Core Principles of the Arachnoiditis Diet Plan

Living with arachnoiditis means navigating symptoms that are heavily influenced by inflammation and nerve function. Although there is no cure for this chronic condition, diet can play a significant role in dampening inflammation and supporting nervous system health. Embracing foundational principles in dietary habits provides a structured, reliable approach that can empower individuals to take greater control of their well-being. This chapter distills the evidence-based core principles of the Arachnoiditis Diet Plan, offering real-world strategies that align with both research and daily practicality.

Emphasis on Whole, Minimally Processed Foods

The first and perhaps most important principle is ***prioritizing whole, minimally processed foods***. These foods such as fresh vegetables, fruits, legumes, nuts, seeds, and unrefined grains form the backbone of many anti-inflammatory diets. Processing often strips foods of beneficial fiber, micronutrients, and phytochemicals that naturally regulate inflammation and support the body's self-repair mechanisms. By contrast, whole foods retain their nutritional complexity and help modulate blood sugar responses, strengthen the gut microbiome, and provide antioxidants critical for nerve protection.

For example, compare a bowl of brown rice and steamed broccoli with a frozen meal high in preservatives and sodium. The whole food meal delivers vitamins, minerals, and phytochemicals without the burden of additives, making it far preferable in any plan targeting chronic inflammation. Individuals with arachnoiditis often notice improved energy and reduced pain flare-ups when meals are based on simple, recognizable ingredients.

Practical ways to shift towards whole, minimally processed foods include:

- Shopping mainly around the perimeter of the grocery store, where fresh produce, meats, and dairy are usually found.
- Cooking meals at home from scratch when possible.
- Reading ingredient lists to choose products with the fewest additives and unpronounceable substances.

By filling your plate with foods as close as possible to their natural form, you create a dietary environment that is inherently more anti-inflammatory and nerve-friendly.

Prioritization of Anti-Inflammatory Nutrients (Omega-3s and Flavonoids)

Not all nutrients impact inflammation equally. Certain anti-inflammatory compounds strongly support nervous system health and can moderate the immune response underlying arachnoiditis symptoms.

Omega-3 fatty acids, abundant in fatty fish (like salmon, sardines, and mackerel), flaxseed, chia seeds, and walnuts, possess a well-documented capacity to reduce systemic inflammation and improve nerve membrane function. They are known to shift the balance from pro-inflammatory to anti-inflammatory compounds within the body, offering protection for nerve cells and the delicate arachnoid tissue that encapsulates them.

Flavonoids, a diverse group of plant-derived antioxidants, also deserve special mention. Found in berries, cherries, citrus fruits, onions, leafy greens, and teas, these compounds help neutralize harmful free radicals, reduce oxidative stress on nerves, and support a balanced immune response. Clinical research highlights that diets rich in flavonoid-containing foods are associated with lower inflammatory markers and improved symptoms in various chronic pain conditions..

Actionable steps to integrate anti-inflammatory nutrients include:

- Eating at least two servings of fatty fish per week, or opting for plant-based omega-3 sources if vegetarian or vegan.
- Adding a handful of berries or a citrus fruit to breakfast or snacks.
- Including colorful, leafy vegetables at lunch and dinner.
- Using herbs and spices (such as turmeric and ginger) regularly not just for flavor, but for their anti-inflammatory benefits.

Through intentional food choices, it is possible to harness the natural healing properties found in key nutrients and help regulate the biological processes underlying pain and inflammation.

Reducing Intake of Added Sugars, saturated Fats, and Food Additives

Conversely, certain dietary components can fuel inflammatory pathways and worsen nerve sensitivity. The modern diet is often overloaded with added sugars, saturated and trans fats, and a variety of artificial additives, all implicated in increased inflammation and metabolic stress.

Added sugars, found in sodas, pastries, sweetened cereals, and many processed foods, cause rapid spikes in blood glucose and insulin levels. These fluctuations not only stress the nervous system but also promote low-grade inflammation throughout the body. Saturated fats, commonly sourced from fatty cuts of red meat, butter, and many store-bought snacks, disrupt cellular membranes and can exacerbate inflammatory activity, particularly when they crowd out healthier unsaturated fats.

Food additives and preservatives, including artificial flavors, colors, and emulsifiers, can compromise gut health and potentially increase immune reactivity in susceptible individuals. This is particularly relevant for those with chronic conditions like arachnoiditis, where immune dysfunction is already present.

To reduce harmful ingredients, try the following:

- Replace sugary drinks with water infused with fruit slices or herbal teas.
- Moderate consumption of fatty meats, choosing fish, poultry, or plant-based proteins more often.
- Read labels to avoid foods with added sugars, trans fats, and unfamiliar additives.
- Prepare simple snacks such as nuts, seeds, and fresh fruit—in place of packaged crackers or granola bars.

Incremental shifts away from foods that fuel inflammation can have a compounding effect, leading to steadier energy, improved gut function, and fewer pain flare-ups.

Adequate hydration and electrolyte management

Water is often overlooked in anti-inflammatory nutrition, yet hydration is fundamental for cellular repair and nerve health. Chronic dehydration can exacerbate nerve pain, slow the clearance of inflammatory byproducts, and disrupt electrolyte balance potentially increasing the risk of muscle cramps or spasms common in arachnoiditis.

Electrolytes, such as sodium, potassium, magnesium, and calcium, are essential for nerve signal transmission and muscle function. Imbalances may worsen neuropathic symptoms or contribute to fatigue. Maintaining adequate hydration and balanced electrolytes is particularly critical for those managing chronic pain, as some medications or decreased physical activity may increase risk for dehydration or deficiencies.

Practical hydration tips include:

- Aim for at least 6–8 cups of fluids daily, adjusting based on individual needs, weather, and activity level.
- Include watery foods such as cucumbers, lettuce, watermelon, and soups.
- If using sports drinks for electrolyte replacement, opt for low-sugar versions or homemade mixtures using water, a splash of fruit juice, and a pinch of sea salt.

- Monitor for signs of dehydration, such as dark urine or headache, and adjust intake accordingly.

Ensuring proper hydration and electrolyte balance helps minimize cramps, supports regular digestion, and creates an internal environment more favorable for nerve recovery.

Timing and Consistency of Meal Routines for Nerve Stabilization

Finally, the pattern and timing of meals are as significant as the foods themselves. Irregular eating, skipped meals, or large, infrequent intakes can destabilize blood sugar, leading to increased nerve excitability and fluctuating energy levels. For individuals with nerve pain, stable blood sugar and routine nourishment help prevent pain flares and support steady moods.

Arachnoiditis sufferers benefit from regular, well-spaced meals and snacks that deliver a combination of complex carbohydrates, lean proteins, and healthy fats. This approach ensures a sustained release of glucose, minimizes spikes in inflammatory markers, and supports optimal nerve signaling.

To implement this principle:

- Eat meals at consistent times each day, aiming for 3 main meals and 1–2 snacks depending on hunger and activity.

- Pair carbohydrates with protein or fat (e.g., apple with nut butter) to slow sugar absorption and stabilize energy.
- Avoid extended fasting (unless medically advised) as this can increase pain sensitivity for some people with chronic nerve conditions.

Keeping meal times regular and balanced helps the nervous system remain calm and reduces the risk of blood sugar-driven pain episodes or fatigue.

The core principles of the Arachnoiditis Diet Plan collectively provide a framework to help reduce inflammation, protect nerve tissue, and stabilize energy levels on a daily basis. They are rooted in both modern research and practical experience from individuals who have learned to manage chronic pain more effectively. Adopting these dietary strategies does not require perfection. Progress is made one thoughtful choice at a time.

Whether you are new to anti-inflammatory eating or seeking to refine an established routine, begin by focusing on one or two principles at a time. For example, start by adding an extra serving of leafy greens to your day or swapping out a sugary snack for mixed nuts and berries. These changes build resilience and give the body the resources it needs for better management of arachnoiditis symptoms.

Foods to Include for Nerve Pain Support

Choosing foods strategically can have a powerful impact on inflammation and nerve pain management, particularly for conditions like arachnoiditis. While the previous chapter established the foundational rules of the Arachnoiditis Diet Plan, this chapter highlights specific foods to prioritize.

Each of these selections is supported by robust research for its role in reducing inflammation, protecting nerves, or supporting overall nervous system health. By incorporating these foods into your daily routine, you create a nutritional environment that works with your body's healing mechanisms.

Fatty Cold-Water Fish: Omega-3 Powerhouses

Fatty fish; such as salmon, sardines, and mackerel—are among the most well-studied foods for supporting nerve health and reducing chronic inflammation. These fish are especially rich in omega-3 polyunsaturated fatty acids, namely EPA (eicosapentaenoic acid) and DHA (docosahexaenoic acid). Omega-3s are known to hinder the production of inflammatory molecules called cytokines and eicosanoids, which play a significant role in the escalation and persistence of nerve pain in chronic conditions like arachnoiditis.

In practical terms, regular consumption of fatty fish has been shown to reduce not just systemic inflammation but also specific markers linked to neuropathic pain. Some clinical studies have found that higher intakes of omega-3s are associated with decreased pain intensity, reduced nerve damage markers, and improvements in quality of life for people with chronic pain disorders. For those seeking non-fish sources, certain algae-based supplements can provide EPA and DHA, but fish itself also brings protein and selenium, two important co-factors for nerve repair.

To get these benefits:

- Aim for at least two servings of fatty fish per week.
- Enjoy grilled salmon with lemon and dill as a main course.
- Add sardines to salads for a quick, nutrient-dense lunch.
- Mackerel can be enjoyed grilled or broiled alongside steamed vegetables.

Leafy Greens and Cruciferous Vegetables: Micronutrient and Phytonutrient Foundations

Leafy greens such as spinach, kale, Swiss chard, and arugula, as well as cruciferous vegetables like broccoli, Brussels sprouts, and cauliflower, are nutritional standouts for nerve pain support. These vegetables are concentrated sources of vitamins C, K, and E, as well as folate and several essential minerals. All of these play roles in nerve function, neurotransmitter production, and anti-inflammatory processes.

Cruciferous vegetables, in particular, are high in sulforaphane, a compound that activates the body's antioxidant defense systems and has demonstrated neuroprotective effects in preclinical studies. Both leafy greens and crucifers are also loaded with fiber, which supports gut health. A healthy gut microbiome, in turn, is associated with lower systemic inflammation and improved nerve signaling.

Simple ways to include these vegetables:

- Add a handful of baby spinach or kale to smoothies for a mild, nutrient-rich boost.
- Steam broccoli or Brussels sprouts and toss them with a drizzle of olive oil and a sprinkle of pepper.

- Make salads with a mix of dark leafy greens and cruciferous vegetables, topped with seeds or nuts for extra crunch.
- Sauté Swiss chard, garlic, and lemon as a flavorful side dish.

Berries, Cherries, and Citrus Fruits: Antioxidant-Rich Choices

Oxidative stress is a significant contributor to nerve injury and chronic pain. Berries (such as blueberries, strawberries, blackberries), cherries, and citrus fruits (including oranges, grapefruits, and lemons) are exceptional sources of antioxidants—compounds that neutralize free radicals and help prevent oxidative damage to nerve tissues.

Many of these fruits are rich in flavonoids and vitamin C, both of which have strong anti-inflammatory properties and support the body's natural pain-moderation pathways. Research has demonstrated that high intake of flavonoid-rich berries is associated with improved nerve resilience, reduced markers of oxidative stress, and decreased overall inflammation. Cherries, especially tart cherries, have been noted for their ability to dampen pain signals and reduce delayed-onset muscle soreness, making them valuable for people whose pain may be worsened by physical activity.

Tips for incorporating these fruits:

- Blend berries into smoothies for breakfast or snacks.
- Add fresh citrus slices to water for enhanced hydration and flavor.
- Top oatmeal or yogurt with a medley of chopped berries and cherries.
- Enjoy an orange or grapefruit as a refreshing, antioxidant-rich dessert.

Whole Grains: Steady Energy and Inflammation Control

Whole grains such as quinoa, brown rice, and millet provide much more than just carbohydrate energy. Unlike refined grains, these whole varieties retain their bran, germ, and endosperm, delivering a full spectrum of nutrition including B vitamins, magnesium, zinc, and fiber. Each of these nutrients supports optimal nerve function and helps control inflammation by regulating immune activity and stabilizing blood sugar.

Magnesium, found abundantly in quinoa and brown rice, is especially relevant because it has been shown to calm nerve excitability and decrease pain transmission. A diet rich in whole grains also contributes to a healthier gut microbiome and steady energy levels throughout the day, which can be critical for those with chronic pain.

Ways to add whole grains to your diet:

- Use quinoa or brown rice as the base for grain bowls with roasted veggies and fish.
- Prepare millet as a side dish with herbs and olive oil.
- Switch out white rice or pasta for their whole grain versions in your favorite recipes.
- Make porridge or breakfast bowls using cooked quinoa, millet, or brown rice, topped with fruit and seeds.

Spices with Anti-Inflammatory Properties: Small Amounts, Big Impact

Sometimes, the most powerful anti-inflammatory compounds come from the smallest ingredients. Spices like turmeric, ginger, and cinnamon have robust scientific backing for their ability to blunt inflammation and moderate pain pathways.

Turmeric contains curcumin, a compound shown to inhibit pro-inflammatory molecules and potentially reduce neuropathic pain symptoms. Both ginger and cinnamon are recognized for their antioxidant effects, and ginger, in particular, has demonstrated benefits for pain and nausea—making it helpful for some of the symptoms seen with chronic nerve inflammation.

Easy tips for adding anti-inflammatory spices:

- Stir turmeric and ginger into soups, stews, and curries for warmth and flavor.

- Add ground cinnamon to oatmeal, smoothies, or even savory pilafs.
- Brew a tea of fresh ginger and turmeric for a calming beverage.
- Use these spices in salad dressings or marinades for an extra anti-inflammatory kick.

Making These Foods Part of Your Routine

Integrating these foods into your week does not require a drastic overhaul of your eating patterns. It's about making intentional choices and small substitutions that reinforce your anti-inflammatory goals:

- Swap processed snacks for a bowl of berries or a handful of nuts and citrus segments.
- Center meals around a serving of fatty fish or a robust mix of beans and leafy greens.
- Choose whole grains for breakfast and sides, crowding out refined grain options.
- Add spices to both familiar and new recipes to boost both flavor and health benefits.

Building familiarity with these foods makes grocery shopping and meal preparation quicker and more intuitive. Batch-cooking a grain or roasting a tray of vegetables ahead of time further streamlines healthy eating, leaving you with easy, pain-supportive options on busy days.

Practical Example: A Sample Day of Anti-Inflammatory Meals

Breakfast

Oatmeal topped with blueberries, sliced almonds, and a dusting of cinnamon.

Lunch

Salad of mixed leafy greens, quinoa, grilled salmon, and a lemon-ginger vinaigrette.

Snack

An orange and a few walnuts.

Dinner

Stir-fried mackerel with broccoli, cauliflower, and snap peas, seasoned with turmeric and garlic.

Dessert

Cherries or a berry-compote with a dollop of Greek yogurt.

Building a nutrition plan for nerve pain relief and inflammation control starts with these five food groups. Fatty cold-water fish provide restorative omega-3s; leafy and cruciferous vegetables nourish with vitamins, minerals, and phytonutrients; berries, cherries, and citrus fruits combat oxidative stress; whole grains deliver steady energy and vital micronutrients; and anti-inflammatory spices give even modest meals a therapeutic edge. Incorporating these foods consistently creates a foundation for better nerve health and overall comfort, making them central to any evidence-based diet for chronic nerve pain support.

Foods and Ingredients to Avoid or Limit

Optimal nutrition for arachnoiditis and nerve pain does not just involve choosing the right foods to support the body, but also requires awareness of which foods and ingredients can undermine progress by promoting inflammation, disrupting nerve health, or aggravating existing symptoms. While the previous chapter outlined foods to prioritize, this chapter focuses on what to avoid or limit as part of a comprehensive anti-inflammatory diet. Awareness and moderation with these foods can play a vital role in reducing flare-ups, stabilizing energy, and supporting long-term wellbeing.

Refined Sugars and Sweetened Beverages

Refined sugars, found in ***table sugar, syrups, candies, baked goods, and sweetened beverages***, are top contributors to increased inflammation. Consuming high amounts of sugar can drive both metabolic stress and chronic inflammatory processes in the body, which may worsen nerve pain and hinder recovery for people with arachnoiditis. Processed sugars, unlike naturally occurring sugars from whole fruits, are metabolized quickly and can cause spikes in blood glucose. This in turn leads to an exaggerated insulin response and the release of pro-inflammatory cytokines.

Sweetened beverages, such as ***sodas, energy drinks, bottled teas, fruit drinks, and "sports" beverages***, are particularly problematic. They offer concentrated sugars absorbed rapidly into the bloodstream, frequently leading to blood sugar swings that can exacerbate neuropathic pain and fatigue. Chronic high sugar intake is associated with higher levels of C-reactive protein (CRP), a marker of inflammation linked to chronic pain disorders.

It's important to check ingredient labels since sugar is often listed under different names, including sucrose, high fructose corn syrup, maltose, dextrose, agave nectar, and many others. If possible, replace sugary drinks with water, herbal teas, or naturally flavored water using citrus or fresh berries. For those with a sweet tooth, opt for whole fruit rather than processed sweets. Not only does this reduce sugar intake, but it also increases fiber consumption, which can further moderate inflammation and improve gut health.

High-sodium processed and packaged snacks

Many snack foods are highly processed and contain significant amounts of sodium as a preservative and flavor enhancer. These include ***potato chips, crackers, packaged***

snack cakes, processed cheeses, canned soups, deli meats, and ready-to-eat meals. Regular consumption of high-sodium foods can disrupt fluid balance, increase blood pressure, and may be a risk factor for elevated inflammation levels.

High sodium intake is linked with vascular dysfunction, which can further compromise nerve and tissue oxygenation in people already struggling with pain and compromised nerve health. Furthermore, excess sodium may affect the immune system, promoting a pro-inflammatory state that can contribute to the chronic pain experienced in arachnoiditis. For individuals managing a chronic pain condition, maintaining a moderate sodium intake is recommended—ideally below 2,300 milligrams per day or as directed by a healthcare provider.

Practical strategies include preparing snacks at home, reading nutritional labels for sodium content, and selecting products labeled as "low sodium" or "no added salt." Substituting packaged snacks with fresh vegetables, plain popcorn, or unsalted nuts can not only lower sodium intake but also provide beneficial micronutrients and fiber.

Fried Foods and Hydrogenated Fats

Fried foods are typically high in unhealthy fats, particularly those prepared using hydrogenated or partially hydrogenated oils. These oils contain trans fats, which are artificially produced fats associated with heightened inflammation, elevated LDL cholesterol, reduced HDL cholesterol, and an increased risk of cardiovascular disease. For those with nerve pain and chronic inflammation, trans fat intake can worsen systemic inflammation and impede the body's ability to heal or manage pain effectively.

Fried foods such as ***French fries, doughnuts, fried chicken, and certain snack*** chips are not only calorie-dense, but their method of preparation often leads to the creation of compounds that can contribute to oxidative stress. Prolonged high heat cooking in vegetable oils, especially those reused in deep fryers, produces advanced glycation end products (AGEs) and oxidized lipids, both of which are implicated in nerve sensitization and inflammatory responses.

To reduce exposure, limit or avoid foods that are battered and deep-fried. Instead, choose cooking methods like baking, roasting, steaming, or air frying. Swap out hydrogenated oils for healthier fats; such as olive oil, avocado oil, and small amounts of coconut oil when preparing meals at home. Opting for "trans fat-free" products and checking for "partially hydrogenated oil" in ingredient lists can also help steer clear of hidden sources.

Artificial preservatives and coloring agents

Packaged and processed foods often contain artificial additives used to extend shelf life, improve appearance, or intensify flavor. Common examples include preservatives like

sodium benzoate, BHA, BHT, nitrates, and nitrites, as well as ***coloring agents such as Red 40, Yellow 5***, and other artificial dyes. Emerging research suggests that some artificial additives may enhance inflammatory pathways or, in sensitive individuals, contribute to immune system over-activation.

Some preservatives are also potentially neurotoxic, and their consumption has been associated with disruptions in gut microbiota and immune function. Since gut health is increasingly recognized as central to inflammation and nervous system health, minimizing exposure to non-essential food additives is a proactive step for those with arachnoiditis. Artificial colors have also been implicated in hypersensitivity reactions in certain individuals, manifesting as headaches or increased pain.

Choose foods with a short, recognizable ingredient list, and minimize intake of brightly colored processed snacks, sweetened cereals, packaged baked goods, and cured meats. When possible, select products labeled as "preservative-free" or "free from artificial colors." Opting for homemade versions of sauces, dressings, and meals further limits exposure to these unnecessary additives.

Excessive alcohol and caffeine intake

Moderation is key with both alcohol and caffeine, two substances that, especially in excess, can exacerbate nerve sensitivity, disrupt sleep, and trigger inflammation.

Excessive alcohol use is associated with direct neurotoxic effects, potentially aggravating existing neuropathic pain and impeding nerve healing. Chronic alcohol consumption increases the production of free radicals and pro-inflammatory mediators, which contribute to the underlying pathophysiology of chronic pain conditions, including arachnoiditis. Alcohol also impairs nutritional absorption, particularly of B vitamins and magnesium, both essential for nerve function and repair.

When it comes to caffeine, moderate intake (up to about 400 milligrams per day, roughly 3-4 cups of coffee for most adults) is generally considered safe for healthy individuals. However, excessive caffeine can lead to heightened pain perception, anxiety, sleep disturbances, and rapid heart rate all of which may worsen pain experiences in individuals with nerve inflammation. Sensitive individuals may find that even less caffeine triggers symptoms, so paying attention to personal tolerance and symptom tracking is key.

Take care to monitor all possible sources of caffeine, including energy drinks, "pre-workout" powders, sodas, chocolate, and some pain relievers. If you notice increased nerve pain, disrupted sleep, or anxiety, consider gradually reducing caffeine intake and exploring non-caffeinated alternatives like herbal teas or warm spiced beverages.

Practical Example: Navigating a Day of Balanced Choices

A typical day often presents common dietary pitfalls, but making mindful alternatives can lead to healthier choices:

- Begin your day with a bowl of overnight oats topped with berries instead of a sugar-sweetened breakfast cereal or pastry. This switch reduces refined sugar and boosts fiber and antioxidants.
- Choose air-popped popcorn or a small handful of unsalted almonds in place of packaged chips or crackers.
- For lunch, select a salad with grilled chicken, olive oil dressing, and plenty of colorful vegetables rather than deli meats piled high on white bread with processed cheese.
- Replace afternoon sodas with herbal tea or sparkling water with a splash of citrus.
- When preparing dinner, bake or grill fish with vegetables rather than deep-frying, and season with herbs and spices instead of relying on processed sauces.
- Limit alcoholic beverages, reserving them for social occasions, and opt for non-alcoholic options more often. Try winding down with a caffeine-free herbal tea in the evening instead of a second coffee or energy drink.

Adjusting your diet for better pain control and inflammation management does not require perfection, but rather persistence and gradual improvement. Each step away from foods that promote inflammation—and towards those that support healing—can make a difference over time. By consciously limiting refined sugars, sodium, fried foods, artificial additives, and excess alcohol or caffeine, you create a more supportive environment for nerve health and overall wellbeing.

Remember that everyone's response to specific foods can vary. Keeping a simple food and symptom diary may help you identify personal triggers or sensitivities and fine-tune your diet accordingly. Working with a healthcare provider or registered dietitian familiar with nerve pain can provide essential guidance on avoiding these problematic foods safely and sustainably.

Meal Planning and Preparation Strategies

Navigating an anti-inflammatory diet for arachnoiditis and nerve pain can seem daunting, especially when busy schedules or fluctuating symptoms make cooking feel overwhelming. A structured approach to meal planning and preparation does more than reduce daily stress; it ensures consistent access to nutrient-rich, nerve-supportive foods and minimizes reliance on last-minute, less optimal choices. In this chapter, you'll find practical frameworks, techniques, and tips for making healthy eating a sustainable part of your lifestyle.

Weekly Meal Template with Breakfast, Lunch, and Dinner Slots

Routine is powerful for those managing chronic nerve pain. A weekly meal template creates predictability, helps balance nutrition across the week, and alleviates decision fatigue. Start by making a simple grid with days of the week as columns and meal times—breakfast, lunch, dinner—as rows.

Within each slot, you can jot down general meal ideas or specific recipes, depending on your preference.

For maximum anti-inflammatory benefit, aim to include:

- ***Diverse color and nutrient variety***: Consider alternating different sources of leafy greens, whole grains, lean proteins (such as salmon, sardines, or plant-based options), and a rotation of berries or citrus.
- ***Flexible "foundation meals"***: Batch-prepped brown rice and roasted vegetables can work as a base for multiple dinners, while overnight oats can serve as both breakfast or a portable snack.
- ***Simple swaps to match your daily needs***: If mornings are rushed, list grab-and-go options (chia pudding with berries, nut butter toast with spinach). Reserve more involved recipes for relaxed evenings.

Here's how one week might look:

Monday:

- *Breakfast*: Oatmeal with flaxseed and blueberries
- *Lunch*: Quinoa salad with roasted vegetables and chickpeas
- *Dinner*: Baked salmon with spinach and brown rice

Tuesday:

- *Breakfast*: Chia pudding with walnuts and cherries
- *Lunch*: Lentil soup with whole-grain toast

- *Dinner*: Stir-fried tofu, broccoli, and red bell pepper on millet

Wednesday:

- *Breakfast*:
  Greek yogurt with sliced almonds and raspberries

- *Lunch*:
  Whole-wheat pita stuffed with hummus, cucumber, and tomato

- *Dinner*:
  Grilled chicken breast with sweet potato and steamed green beans

Thursday:

- *Breakfast*:
  Smoothie with spinach, banana, protein powder, and almond milk

- *Lunch*:
  Brown rice bowl with black beans, corn, avocado, and salsa

- *Dinner*:
  Baked cod with roasted Brussels sprouts and quinoa

Friday:

- *Breakfast*:
  Scrambled eggs with sautéed mushrooms and tomatoes

- *Lunch*:
  Farro salad with arugula, roasted beets, and goat cheese

- *Dinner*:
  Vegetable curry with chickpeas served over brown rice

Saturday:

- *Breakfast*:
  Buckwheat pancakes with fresh strawberries

- *Lunch*:
  Minestrone soup with whole-grain crackers

- *Dinner*:
  Grilled turkey burger with lettuce, tomato, and a side of roasted carrots

Sunday:

- *Breakfast*:
  Overnight oats with chia seeds, apple, and cinnamon

- *Lunch*:
  Spinach and lentil salad with pumpkin seeds and balsamic vinaigrette

- *Dinner*:
  Baked eggplant with tomato sauce and mozzarella, served with quinoa

Relying on a template also allows for easy grocery planning, decreasing the risk of impulse purchases or less supportive meal choices when symptoms flare.

Batch Cooking and Freezer-Friendly Anti-Inflammatory Staples

Batch cooking is a practical approach that allows you to make the most of days when your energy is higher, enabling you to prepare a variety of nutritious meals in advance. By dedicating time to cook in larger quantities, you can create a reserve of healthy options for days when fatigue or pain makes meal preparation more challenging.

In addition to ensuring that wholesome food is always within reach, batch cooking reduces the overall time spent on meal prep, helps with portion control, and decreases the likelihood of turning to takeout or processed snacks during busy or low-energy periods.

Here are some key batch cooking strategies to maximize convenience and nutrition:

1. ***Choose recipes that store and reheat well.*** Focus on dishes such as soups, stews, grain salads, and roasted vegetables, which maintain their flavor, texture, and nutritional value even after freezing and reheating.
2. ***Freeze meals in single or double portions.*** Use freezer-safe containers or reusable silicone bags to

make it easy to grab exactly what you need. This also helps minimize food waste and ensures meals are ready to go.

3. ***Clearly label all containers***. Include the name of the meal and the date it was prepared to help track freshness and simplify meal selection.

Some examples of anti-inflammatory batch and freezer staples include:

1. ***Sweet potato and lentil soup***. This dish is high in fiber, antioxidants, and slow-digesting carbohydrates, which provide sustained energy and support nerve health.
2. ***Roasted turmeric cauliflower and chickpeas***. The combination offers anti-inflammatory spices along with plant-based protein for a nutritious and satisfying meal.
3. ***Blueberry chia seed pudding***. Packed with omega-3 fatty acids, antioxidants, and prebiotic fibers, this option is both nourishing and easy to store.

To begin, try selecting two or three recipes each week specifically for batch cooking. Dedicate a couple of hours, perhaps on the weekend, to preparing and packaging your meals. With several ready-to-eat options available in your freezer, making daily meal decisions becomes simpler and less stressful, supporting your overall health and well-being.

Portion Control Techniques for Energy Management

Portion control plays a crucial role for individuals managing chronic nerve pain. Both overeating and undereating can significantly affect inflammation, blood sugar stability, and overall well-being. Maintaining mindful portions throughout the day can help stabilize energy levels and may reduce post-meal symptoms such as fatigue, discomfort, and mood swings. By adopting effective portion control strategies, individuals can support better pain management and maintain a more balanced lifestyle.

Here are some practical portion control techniques you can incorporate into your daily routine:

1. ***Use smaller plates and bowls***: Smaller dishware helps visually limit serving sizes, making it easier to avoid oversized portions without feeling deprived.
2. ***Pre-portion snacks***: Instead of eating directly from large bags or containers, divide snacks like nuts, berries, or cut vegetables into single-serving containers. This helps prevent mindless eating and makes healthier choices more accessible.
3. ***Structure your plate***: Aim to fill half your plate with non-starchy vegetables, such as leafy greens, broccoli, or bell peppers. Reserve one quarter of your plate for lean protein sources like chicken, fish, tofu, or legumes. Use the remaining quarter for whole grains or

starchy vegetables, such as brown rice, quinoa, or sweet potatoes. This balanced approach can help manage blood sugar and inflammation while keeping you satisfied.

4. ***Eat slowly and pause between bites***: Taking your time with meals allows your body to recognize feelings of fullness, which can prevent overeating. Pausing between bites and chewing thoroughly also aids digestion and enhances mindfulness around eating.
5. ***Portion when batch cooking or freezing***: When preparing meals in bulk, divide food into individual portions before storing. This makes it easier to grab appropriately-sized meals and reduces the temptation to eat more than necessary.
6. ***Tune into hunger and fullness cues***: Pay close attention to your body's signals. Consider keeping a meal and symptom journal to track how varying portion sizes affect your pain levels, energy, and mood throughout the day. This awareness can help you make more informed decisions that support your overall health.

Consistently practicing these techniques, you can foster healthier eating habits and support steady energy, which is especially important when managing chronic nerve pain.

Shopping List Organization by Food Group

An organized shopping list is a fundamental tool for sticking with an anti-inflammatory meal plan. Not only does it streamline your shopping trips, but it also minimizes the chances of purchasing foods that may trigger inflammation or nerve irritation.

The most effective approach categorizes foods by major groups:

Produce:

- Leafy greens (spinach, kale, arugula)
- Cruciferous vegetables (broccoli, cauliflower)
- Berries, cherries, citrus
- Sweet potatoes and other root vegetables

Proteins:

Fresh or frozen salmon, sardines, mackerel

Legumes (lentils, chickpeas, black beans)

Tofu, tempeh

Nuts and seeds (walnuts, chia, flaxseed)

Whole Grains:

- Brown rice
- Quinoa
- Millet

- Steel-cut oats

Pantry Staples:

- Olive oil, avocado oil
- Spices (turmeric, ginger, cinnamon)
- Low-sodium vegetable broth

Dairy/Dairy-Alternatives:

- Unsweetened plant-based milks (almond, oat, coconut)
- Plain Greek yogurt (if tolerated)

This arrangement simplifies shopping and encourages you to focus on nutrient-dense options. Consider keeping a reusable list or a digital checklist to update regularly based on seasonality or recipe needs.

Substitution Guide for Allergen-Friendly Recipe Adjustments

Dietary restrictions, food allergies, or intolerances should not limit your access to anti-inflammatory recipes. Learning simple, reliable substitutions empowers you to safely prepare and enjoy a wide variety of meals—even if avoiding common triggers such as gluten, dairy, eggs, nuts, or soy.

Here are some common swaps that preserve nutrition and flavor:

- ***Instead of wheat***: Use gluten-free grains like quinoa, brown rice, millet, or certified gluten-free oats.

- ***Instead of dairy milk***: Choose unsweetened almond, soy, oat, or coconut milk. If baking, opt for options with a similar fat content to cow's milk for texture.
- ***Instead of eggs***: For binding in baking, use a "flax egg" (1 tablespoon ground flaxseed mixed with 2.5 tablespoons water), mashed banana, or unsweetened applesauce.
- ***Instead of nuts***: Substitute sunflower or pumpkin seeds, or use nut-free seed butters in smoothies and baking.
- ***Instead of soy***: Swap tofu or tempeh for legumes (lentils, chickpeas), or use jackfruit for a pulled texture in savory dishes.

Consider food intolerances, such as sensitivity to nightshades (tomatoes, peppers, eggplant, white potato). In recipes requiring tomatoes, try roasted carrots or pureed pumpkin for a sweet, vibrant alternative. For potatoes, use sweet potatoes or parsnips.

Remember to adjust spices and seasonings as needed, since pre-mixed blends can contain gluten or hidden allergens. Prepare your own anti-inflammatory spice mixes using pure ground turmeric, ginger, cinnamon, and black pepper.

Embracing these meal planning and preparation strategies will not only help you adhere to an anti-inflammatory diet plan but also foster confidence and independence in the kitchen. The next chapter will build on these foundations with concrete strategies for symptom tracking, trigger identification, and navigating dietary challenges as they arise.

Flare-Reduction Strategies Beyond Food Choice

Living with arachnoiditis or chronic nerve pain means managing more than your basic calories and nutrients. While food selection is essential, individuals often notice that their symptoms fluctuate even when eating a healthy, balanced diet. This variability can be linked to a combination of dietary triggers, meal timing, stress levels, and other lifestyle factors. In this chapter, we focus on approaches that extend beyond the standard "what to eat" advice. You'll learn how to pinpoint your personal triggers, harness mindful eating, control blood sugar, and use gentle strategies during flares, forming a comprehensive toolkit for reducing symptom exacerbations.

Identifying and Tracking Dietary Flare Triggers

Everyone's response to food is unique, particularly for those managing complex conditions like arachnoiditis. While some people experience heightened pain shortly after consuming processed foods, others might find seemingly innocuous foods; such as certain fruits or grains, act as triggers. Identifying your individual flare triggers is the first proactive step in controlling symptoms.

A food and symptom diary is a valuable tool for this task. Start by recording everything you eat and drink, including snacks, condiments, and supplements. Alongside each meal entry, note the date, time eaten, and any symptoms that arise such as pain spikes, tingling, digestive changes, or fatigue. Use intensity scales (e.g., 0–10) to give a quantitative sense of symptom fluctuations throughout the day. Over a period of several weeks, patterns often emerge, revealing links between particular foods or ingredients and the onset or worsening of symptoms.

Keep in mind that some reactions may be delayed by several hours or even up to a day, so consider potential lag time when assessing associations. Furthermore, non-dietary factors like stress, changes in physical activity, or sleep quality can confound patterns; recording these alongside meals helps provide context and increases the usefulness of your diary. Many find it helpful to review charts weekly and look for recurring links, such as higher pain levels after consuming a certain type of bread or packaged snack.

If you suspect specific ingredients are problematic, try a methodical approach to elimination and reintroduction. Remove the item for two weeks while observing symptom changes, then gradually reintroduce it. Return of symptoms during reintroduction may confirm a true dietary trigger. Always approach eliminations cautiously and consult with a qualified dietitian or healthcare provider to avoid nutritional gaps and unnecessary restrictions.

Utilizing Low-Glycemic Load Meals for Blood Sugar Stability

Stable blood sugar is crucial for anyone dealing with chronic inflammation and nerve pain. Research has shown that glucose spikes and drops can worsen neuropathic symptoms by fueling cycles of inflammation and oxidative stress within nerve tissues. Highly processed carbohydrates, sugars, and starchy foods (like white bread, pastries, or sweetened beverages) often produce rapid increases and subsequent crashes in blood sugar. This leads not only to overall energy swings, but can potentiate pain flares, especially in susceptible individuals.

Low-glycemic load (GL) meals are designed to minimize these swings. Glycemic load takes into account both the type and quantity of carbohydrate, providing a more accurate prediction of a food's impact on blood sugar compared to glycemic index alone. ***Key strategies for building low-GL meals include***:

- Emphasizing whole grains (such as quinoa, barley, and brown rice) over refined grains.

- Including fiber-rich vegetables, beans, and legumes, which slow glucose absorption.
- Pairing carbohydrate sources with lean protein (e.g., fish, chicken, tofu) and healthy fats (avocado, olive oil) to blunt rapid sugar rises.
- Enjoying whole fruits over juices or dried fruits, and limiting portions of high-sugar items.

A lunch featuring a bowl of lentil soup with leafy greens and a side of wild rice is far less likely to provoke a blood sugar spike than a meal based around white bread sandwiches and soda. By regulating blood sugar, you create a more stable physiological environment, one that reduces the likelihood of immune overreaction and nerve hyperexcitability.

Managing Food Intolerances and Sensitivities

Food intolerances and sensitivities operate differently than classic allergies. Instead of provoking an immediate immune response, intolerances often result in delayed symptoms—ranging from digestive upset to increased pain or fatigue. Inflammation may be subtle, insidious, and uniquely personal; common culprits include lactose, gluten, certain FODMAPs (fermentable carbohydrates), or chemical sensitivities (such as to additives or sulfites).

Those living with nerve pain may find their threshold for food sensitivities is lowered because of an already "activated" immune or nervous system. Increased intestinal permeability ("leaky gut") or alterations in the gut microbiome, both commonly associated with inflammatory disease, can further magnify the impact of these sensitivities on pain signaling and overall well-being.

If you suspect a sensitivity, continue using your food and symptom diary, noting any delayed reactions (up to 72 hours later) such as bloating, headaches, skin flare-ups, or pain intensification. Working with a healthcare professional, targeted elimination diets (such as removing gluten or high-lactose foods) can help clarify whether symptoms improve without certain ingredients.

Be aware that unnecessarily broad elimination—without medical oversight—can lead to nutritional deficiencies or hidden stress. The goal is personalization: remove only those foods that are genuinely problematic, and replace them with equally nutrient-rich alternatives.

Mindful Eating Practices for Symptom Awareness

Eating is often rushed or distracted, particularly on days when pain is intense, but mindful eating offers a gentle yet powerful way to tune into how food affects your body in real-time. Mindful eating means slowing down, paying attention to the sensory experience of eating—taste, texture, aroma—and turning off screens or distractions during meals. This practice not only aids digestion but heightens your awareness of post-meal symptoms, satiety, and potential triggers you might otherwise miss.

Practical steps for mindful eating include:

- Taking a few deep breaths before meals to shift your body into a calm, receptive state (rest-and-digest mode).
- Eating slowly, chewing thoroughly, and savoring flavors.
- Pausing periodically to check in with your body; How is your pain? Does bloating or discomfort start as you eat? Do you feel satisfied, or is there a sensation of fullness or irritation?
- Journaling or mentally noting sensations shortly after eating.

Research indicates that mindful eating supports healthier food choices, improved blood sugar responses, and better recognition of hunger and satiety cues all of which empower individuals to respond proactively to flare warning signs. This self-awareness builds your understanding of which foods and eating habits truly support your healing.

Use of Gentle Herbal Teas and Broths During Exacerbations

Despite the best planning, symptom flares can still happen. During these episodes, regular solid meals might feel unappealing or even intolerable. In such moments, gentle herbal teas and nourishing broths can provide comfort, hydration, and mild anti-inflammatory benefits, without further irritating the digestive or nervous system.

Herbal teas such as ginger, chamomile, and rooibos are well-tolerated by most and contain bioactive compounds with mild anti-inflammatory and soothing effects. Ginger is notable for calming nausea and improving gut motility; chamomile has mild sedative and antispasmodic actions; while rooibos adds natural antioxidants. Sipping these warm liquids can also promote muscle relaxation and a sense of calm during stressful flares.

Homemade vegetable or bone broths are another time-tested option. Rich in minerals and amino acids, broths provide hydration and a gentle delivery of nutrients at times when heavier meals are not tolerated. You can further tailor these with anti-inflammatory additions for instance, a bay leaf, parsley, or turmeric root added during simmering. Individuals with food sensitivities should use simple, clear broths and avoid high-salt or heavily seasoned commercial options, which can provoke symptoms in sensitive individuals.

When using any herbal remedy, proceed cautiously. Although generally safe, it's wise to check for possible allergies or interactions with medications, and always consult with your healthcare provider if unsure.

Beyond what you put on your plate, these flare-reduction strategies offer a more nuanced and individualized approach to managing chronic nerve pain and inflammation. Tracking your unique dietary triggers and intolerances, stabilizing blood sugar, practicing mindful eating, and turning to gentle herbal teas and broths when needed, all add extra layers of support to your anti-inflammatory diet plan. As you experiment with these methods, remember that every body is different. With time and attentive observation, you'll be better equipped to minimize flares and reclaim more symptom-free days.

Simple Recipes for Nerve Pain Support

Adopting a diet rich in anti-inflammatory foods is a practical way to help manage nerve pain, especially for individuals with arachnoiditis or similar conditions. This chapter introduces easy-to-prepare recipes carefully chosen for their ingredients' nerve-supporting and inflammation-fighting qualities. These recipes are designed to fit into everyday routines, with a focus on whole foods, high-fiber grains, lean proteins, and powerful antioxidant sources.

Quinoa and Spinach Breakfast Bowl

Ingredients:

- 3/4 cup cooked quinoa
- 1 handful fresh spinach
- 1 soft-boiled egg or 1/2 sliced avocado
- 1 tablespoon pumpkin seeds
- 1 teaspoon olive oil
- Black pepper, to taste

Instructions:

1. Place warm cooked quinoa in a bowl.
2. Top with fresh spinach, a soft-boiled egg (or sliced avocado), and pumpkin seeds.
3. Drizzle with olive oil and sprinkle with black pepper.
4. Serve immediately for a nutrient-rich breakfast.

Blueberry Chia Seed Pudding

Ingredients:

- 3 tablespoons chia seeds
- 1 cup unsweetened almond milk
- 1/2 cup mashed blueberries

Instructions:

1. In a bowl or jar, mix chia seeds, almond milk, and mashed blueberries.
2. Stir well and refrigerate overnight.
3. In the morning, stir again and enjoy as a breakfast or snack.

Omega-3 Rich Salmon and Broccoli Sheet Pan Dinner

Ingredients:

- 1 salmon fillet
- 2 cups broccoli florets
- 1 tablespoon olive oil
- Black pepper, to taste
- 2–3 lemon slices

Instructions:

1. Preheat the oven to 400°F (205°C).
2. Arrange salmon fillet and broccoli florets on a baking sheet.
3. Drizzle with olive oil and season with black pepper.
4. Top salmon with lemon slices.
5. Roast for 15–20 minutes or until salmon is cooked through and broccoli is tender.

Roasted Turmeric Cauliflower and Chickpeas

Ingredients:

- 2 cups cauliflower florets
- 1 can (15 oz) chickpeas, rinsed and drained
- 1 tablespoon olive oil
- 1 teaspoon turmeric
- Pinch black pepper
- Salt, to taste

Instructions:

1. Preheat the oven to 425°F (220°C).
2. In a bowl, toss cauliflower and chickpeas with olive oil, turmeric, black pepper, and salt.
3. Spread on a baking sheet and roast for 25 minutes, until golden and crispy.

Sweet Potato and Lentil Soup

Ingredients:

- 1 onion, chopped
- 2 cloves garlic, minced
- 2 medium sweet potatoes, diced
- 1 cup dried lentils, rinsed
- 2 carrots, chopped
- 4 cups low-sodium vegetable broth
- 1 teaspoon cumin
- Salt and pepper, to taste
- 2 tablespoons chopped parsley (for garnish)

Instructions:

1. In a large pot, sauté onion and garlic until fragrant.
2. Add sweet potatoes, lentils, and carrots. Stir to combine.
3. Pour in vegetable broth and add cumin, salt, and pepper.
4. Bring to a boil, then simmer until vegetables and lentils are tender (20–25 minutes).
5. Top with chopped parsley before serving.

Berry Almond Overnight Oats

Ingredients:

- 1/2 cup rolled oats
- 1 tablespoon almond butter
- 1 cup unsweetened milk (dairy or plant-based)
- 1/2 cup mixed berries

Instructions:

1. In a jar or airtight container, combine oats, almond butter, milk, and berries.
2. Stir well, cover, and refrigerate overnight.
3. Stir again in the morning and enjoy.

Lemon Garlic Sautéed Greens

Ingredients:

- 2 cups leafy greens (kale, Swiss chard, or spinach), chopped
- 1 tablespoon olive oil
- 2 cloves garlic, minced
- Juice of 1/2 lemon

Instructions:

1. Heat olive oil in a skillet over medium heat.
2. Add garlic and cook until fragrant.
3. Add greens and sauté until just wilted.
4. Squeeze lemon juice over the greens and serve.

Wild Rice and Vegetable Stir-Fry

Ingredients:

- 1 cup wild rice, cooked
- 1 bell pepper, sliced
- 1 carrot, sliced
- 1 cup snap peas
- 1 cup mushrooms, sliced
- 1 tablespoon olive or avocado oil
- 1 tablespoon low-sodium tamari or soy sauce

Instructions:

1. Cook wild rice according to package directions.
2. Heat oil in a skillet or wok.
3. Add vegetables and stir-fry until crisp-tender.
4. Add cooked wild rice and tamari, stirring to combine.
5. Serve warm.

Ginger-Spiced Pumpkin Soup

Ingredients:

- 3 cups peeled, cubed pumpkin (or 2 cups canned pumpkin puree)
- 1 onion, chopped
- 2 cloves garlic, minced
- 1 tablespoon fresh ginger, grated
- 3 cups low-sodium broth
- Salt and pepper, to taste
- 1/4 cup Greek yogurt (optional, for garnish)
- 1 tablespoon chopped chives (optional)

Instructions:

1. In a pot, sauté onion, garlic, and ginger until soft.
2. Add pumpkin and broth. Bring to a boil.
3. Simmer until the pumpkin is soft (about 15–20 minutes).
4. Blend soup until smooth. Season to taste.
5. Garnish with Greek yogurt and chives if desired.

Grilled Mackerel with Herbed Quinoa

Ingredients:

- 2 mackerel fillets
- 1 lemon, sliced
- 1 tablespoon fresh rosemary or thyme
- 1 cup quinoa, cooked
- 2 tablespoons chopped parsley, mint, or basil
- 1 tablespoon olive oil
- Juice of 1/2 lemon

Instructions:

1. Preheat the grill. Season mackerel with lemon slices and herbs.
2. Grill fillets for 3–4 minutes per side, until cooked.
3. In a bowl, mix cooked quinoa with herbs, olive oil, and a squeeze of lemon.
4. Serve mackerel over herbed quinoa.

Mixed Berry Anti-Inflammatory Smoothie

Ingredients:

- 1 cup mixed berries (blueberries, blackberries, raspberries)
- 1/2 banana
- 1 small handful spinach
- 1 tablespoon ground flaxseed
- 1 cup unsweetened milk or kefir

Instructions:

1. Place all ingredients in a blender.
2. Blend until smooth.
3. Pour into a glass and enjoy.

Walnut and Flaxseed Energy Bites

Ingredients:

- 1 cup walnuts
- 1/2 cup rolled oats
- 2 tablespoons flaxseed
- 1/2 cup pitted dates

Instructions:

1. In a food processor, combine all ingredients.
2. Process until mixture is sticky and holds together.
3. Roll into small balls and refrigerate.

Turmeric Chicken Lettuce Wraps

Ingredients:

- 2 chicken breasts, thinly sliced
- 1 tablespoon olive oil
- 1 teaspoon turmeric
- 1/2 teaspoon cumin
- Pinch black pepper
- 8 large butter lettuce leaves
- 1/2 cup shredded carrots
- 1/2 cup cucumber, sliced
- 2 tablespoons tahini sauce

Instructions:

1. In a bowl, toss chicken with olive oil, turmeric, cumin, and black pepper.
2. Sauté chicken in a skillet until cooked through.
3. Place chicken, carrots, and cucumber in lettuce leaves.
4. Drizzle with tahini sauce and serve.

Cinnamon Apple Compote

Ingredients:

- 3 apples, peeled and diced
- 1/2 teaspoon cinnamon
- 2 tablespoons water
- Juice of 1/2 lemon

Instructions:

1. In a saucepan, combine apples, cinnamon, water, and lemon juice.
2. Cook over medium heat until the apples are soft (10–15 minutes).
3. Serve warm over yogurt or chia pudding.

Avocado-Tomato Salad with Fresh Basil

Ingredients:

- 1 ripe avocado, cubed
- 1 cup cherry tomatoes, halved
- 1/4 cup fresh basil leaves
- 1 tablespoon extra-virgin olive oil
- 1 teaspoon balsamic vinegar

Instructions:

1. In a bowl, combine avocado, tomatoes, and basil.
2. Drizzle with olive oil and balsamic vinegar.
3. Toss gently and serve as a side or light lunch.

Tips for Incorporating Nerve-Supportive Recipes

To get the most benefit from these recipes, consider these practical strategies:

- Rotate the main types of protein (fish, legumes, poultry, and seeds) during the week to encourage nutritional variety and balanced omega-3 intake.
- Batch-cook grain bases or soups to freeze in single servings for convenience.
- Prep vegetables in advance to speed up meal assembly.
- Vary herbs and spices, emphasizing those shown to support anti-inflammatory pathways, such as turmeric, ginger, garlic, and cinnamon.

Use these recipes as templates swap similar seasonal vegetables or proteins to maintain nutrient diversity and enjoyment.

With this set of simple recipes at your fingertips, healthy eating for nerve pain support can become a delicious daily habit. Each recipe is designed to reduce inflammation, promote nerve stability, and supply long-lasting energy all important for individuals managing arachnoiditis and chronic neuropathic pain.

Supplementation and Supportive Nutrients

When managing arachnoiditis and chronic nerve pain, a well-structured anti-inflammatory diet forms the foundation of care. Yet, even the most mindful meal plans may leave gaps for nutrients crucial to nerve and immune system health. This is where thoughtful supplementation paired with guidance from healthcare providers can play a supportive role. In this chapter, you'll find evidence-based guidance on which supplements are most often helpful, which to approach with caution, and how to personalize your approach for the best results.

Fish Oil and Vegan Omega-3 Alternatives

Omega-3 fatty acids are essential fats that possess potent anti-inflammatory properties. They are well-known for supporting not only heart and cognitive health, but also for their roles in nerve function and pain modulation. Most notably, omega-3s can contribute to reducing the inflammatory processes implicated in nerve pain conditions like arachnoiditis.

Fish oil is the classic source of two vital long-chain omega-3s: EPA (eicosapentaenoic acid) and DHA (docosahexaenoic acid). These are found abundantly in cold-water fatty fish such as salmon, sardines, and mackerel. For individuals who do not consume fish, either due to dietary preference or allergies, quality vegan alternatives are available. Algal oil, derived from marine algae, is especially promising since it naturally contains DHA and, in many products, EPA as well. This makes algal oil an effective plant-based substitute with similar physiological impacts as fish oil.

Including omega-3 supplements may be especially beneficial when dietary intake of fatty fish is low, or when inflammation is persistent. For newcomers, a typical starting dose ranges from 1000–2000 mg of combined EPA and DHA daily, though doses should ultimately be discussed with a healthcare provider to tailor recommendations and minimize risks, like potential interactions with blood-thinning medications.

Vitamin D and Magnesium for Nerve Health

Vitamin D is often referred to as the "sunshine vitamin" because it is produced in response to sunlight exposure. Despite this, deficiency remains widespread, especially among people living in northern climates or those with limited sun exposure. For individuals with chronic nerve pain, vitamin D deserves special attention: Low levels have been associated with increased pain perception, worsened nerve health, and dysregulated immune responses.

Supplementing with vitamin D is common, and simple blood tests can reveal deficiency and guide appropriate dosing. Maintenance needs vary, but many adults benefit from daily supplementation in the range of 1000 to 2000 IU, especially if baseline levels are insufficient.. However, due to the risk of accumulation and toxicity, doses above 4000 IU daily should not be used unless prescribed and monitored by a healthcare professional.

Magnesium is another critical nutrient for nerve function. It helps regulate neurotransmitters, calm overexcited nerve cells, and may reduce neuropathic pain intensity. Many people do not meet magnesium requirements through food alone, particularly if diets are low in leafy greens, nuts, seeds, and whole grains. Supplementing with magnesium glycinate or magnesium citrate is generally well-tolerated and absorbed magnesium oxide, in contrast, has a higher likelihood of causing digestive upset.

To support nerve health, a typical dose of magnesium ranges from 200 to 400 mg daily, usually taken with food. Start at the lower end and adjust as tolerated, since excessive intake can result in diarrhea or, in rare cases, affect heart rhythm. Individuals with kidney problems should consult their doctor before increasing magnesium through diet or supplements to avoid complications.

Alpha-lipoic acid and Acetyl-L-Carnitine Supplements

Alpha-lipoic acid (ALA) is a powerful antioxidant that plays several roles in cellular energy production and the neutralization of free radicals. It has gained attention for its potential in relieving symptoms of neuropathic pain, particularly among people with diabetes, though its effects may also extend to other types of nerve damage as seen in arachnoiditis. Clinical studies suggest that ALA supplementation may reduce pain and improve nerve conduction by diminishing inflammation and oxidative stress.

Common dosing protocols for ALA in studies range from 300 to 600 mg daily, typically divided across one or two doses. Oral supplementation is most practical for home use, though some clinical trials use intravenous forms under medical supervision.

Acetyl-L-carnitine (ALC) is another supportive compound. As an amino acid derivative, ALC is involved in mitochondrial energy production and has demonstrated positive effects in enhancing nerve regeneration and reducing nerve pain. Supplementation may be especially helpful for older adults or those with deficits due to chronic illness. Typical daily dosages range from 500 to 2000 mg, divided into two doses, but higher doses should only be used under medical advice due to the possibility of side effects such as mild agitation or gastrointestinal symptoms.

As always, discuss the use of these supplements with your provider since they may interact with specific prescription medications or underlying medical conditions.

Cautions Regarding Unchecked Herbal Products

While herbs and botanicals are sometimes considered "natural," their use in pain management must be approached with care. Herbal supplements are regulated differently than conventional medicines and may vary widely in quality, potency, and purity. Some may interact dangerously with prescription medications or trigger allergic reactions.

For example, common nerve pain remedies like St. John's Wort or kava have been documented to interfere with liver enzymes that process many medications, potentially leading to toxicity or reduced effectiveness of other treatments. Similarly, some herbal blends can contain undisclosed ingredients or contaminants, creating unnecessary risks.

<u>If you're considering herbal supplements, it is important to:</u>

1. Seek products tested for quality by independent organizations when possible (look for USP, NSF, or ConsumerLab certifications).
2. Avoid combination or "proprietary blend" products with poorly defined ingredient lists.

3. Inform your healthcare provider of all herbal supplements you are taking to avoid unwanted interactions.

Herbal teas, when used in moderation and clearly labeled, are generally less risky, but even these should be disclosed if you're taking prescription medicines or scheduled for procedures.

Consulting Healthcare Providers for Individualized Supplementation

Dietary supplements can be valuable allies in a holistic approach to managing nerve pain and reducing inflammation. However, the optimal regimen varies based on your unique health status, symptoms, and the medications you may be taking. Self-prescribing supplements can lead to nutrient excesses, drug interactions, or missed opportunities for diagnosing underlying deficiencies that require tailored treatment.

Here's how you can work with your healthcare team to maximize benefits and minimize risks:

1. Before starting any new supplement, discuss your plans with a registered dietitian, pharmacist, or physician familiar with your condition.
2. Ask about laboratory tests to assess baseline levels of vitamin D, magnesium, or other relevant nutrients.

3. Provide a complete list of all supplements and medications you use (including over-the-counter herbs or vitamins) at each clinic visit.
4. If you experience new symptoms or side effects, report these promptly, as they could relate to supplement use.
5. Re-evaluate your supplement plan every six to twelve months to ensure it remains aligned with your evolving health needs.

By taking a collaborative and informed approach, you can safely incorporate supplements that reinforce the foundation established by dietary changes. Remember, supplements are just a supplementary tool, not a substitute for nutrient-rich food or comprehensive medical care.

Making sense of supplementation can feel overwhelming amidst the complexities of chronic nerve pain. By focusing on well-researched options—such as omega-3s, vitamin D, magnesium, alpha-lipoic acid, and acetyl-L-carnitine you can support the body's ability to manage inflammation and protect nerve health. At the same time, maintaining a healthy skepticism toward unverified herbal products and seeking advice from knowledgeable healthcare providers safeguards both your progress and well-being.

Integrating targeted supplements with a foundational anti-inflammatory diet and coordinated professional guidance sets the stage for meaningful, long-term improvements in your journey with arachnoiditis and nerve pain.

Long-Term Diet Sustainability and Lifestyle Integration

For anyone living with arachnoiditis and chronic nerve pain, adopting an anti-inflammatory diet marks the start of an ongoing journey, one that is most successful when built for the long haul. Integrating these dietary changes into your lifestyle is not just about what you eat, but about creating habits, setting achievable milestones, preparing for real-world situations, and recognizing the importance of support and education along the way. In this chapter, you'll find key strategies to help make your dietary changes stick and become an empowering, sustainable part of your everyday life.

Setting Realistic Goals for Dietary Transition

A sustainable dietary change begins with realistic, achievable goals tailored to your current habits and lifestyle. Rather than aiming to overhaul your diet overnight, focus on gradual yet consistent adjustments. This might involve replacing sugary breakfast cereals with a whole grain option, adding one extra serving of vegetables each day, or swapping fried snacks for nutrient-dense alternatives. Research shows that incremental dietary changes are more likely to become permanent, as they allow both your taste preferences and household routines time to adapt.

Setting SMART (Specific, Measurable, Achievable, Relevant, Time-bound) goals helps transform vague intentions into actionable steps. For example:

Specific: "I will prepare home-cooked dinners at least four days per week."

Measurable: "I will include a serving of leafy greens in my lunch every weekday."

Achievable: "I will choose water or unsweetened herbal tea instead of soda once daily."

Relevant: "These changes support my goal to reduce inflammation and manage pain."

Time-bound: "I will reassess my progress in two weeks."

Writing down your goals or sharing them with a supportive family member or care provider can further boost accountability and motivation.

Techniques for Eating Out and Social Events

Eating outside the home can seem challenging when following an anti-inflammatory diet, but with preparation, it's entirely feasible and pleasurable. Start by researching restaurant menus online ahead of time to identify dishes that align with your dietary approach. Many restaurants now offer gluten-free, plant-forward, or explicitly anti-inflammatory menu options. Don't hesitate to call ahead and ask about ingredient swaps or food preparations.

When attending social events or family gatherings, consider these strategies:

1. Eat a small, healthy snack beforehand to avoid arriving overly hungry.
2. Offer to bring a dish you know meets your dietary requirements, such as a colorful salad or a batch of roasted vegetables.
3. Scan the buffet or dinner table, prioritizing whole food options like lean proteins, salads, legumes, and fruit.
4. Practice polite assertiveness: simply let your host know you have specific dietary needs focusing on reducing inflammation and managing health. Most hosts will appreciate the information given in advance.
5. If you do indulge in less optimal choices, focus on moderation, mindful enjoyment, and resume your usual patterns at the next meal.

These approaches help prevent anxiety around eating out and make socializing enjoyable rather than stressful.

Managing Setbacks and Maintaining Motivation

Setbacks are an inevitable part of long-term lifestyle change. There will be days when pain, fatigue, or a busy schedule disrupts your best intentions. What matters most is your response and see these moments as opportunities for learning rather than reasons for discouragement.

<u>**To navigate setbacks:**</u>

- Reflect on triggers. Was there a specific stressor, event, or barrier?
- Reframe your self-talk. Replace "I blew my diet" with "I faced a challenge and can try again tomorrow."
- Plan for the future. Troubleshoot what you can do differently next time, whether that's preparing food in advance or reaching out for support.

Motivation ebbs and flows, but building habits around your goals helps them persist. Keeping a food and symptom journal serves as a powerful reminder of progress and the positive changes you're fostering. Celebrating small wins like finding a new go-to recipe or experiencing a pain-free day is key for long-term forward momentum.

It's also helpful to revisit your "why." Whether it's reducing pain, enhancing mobility, or simply feeling more in control, clarifying your deepest reasons for choosing this path can reignite motivation during tougher times.

Tracking Symptom Changes and Diet Effectiveness

Regular assessment of symptoms and dietary changes is vital for understanding what's working and identifying areas for further refinement. **Begin by keeping a simple journal, noting**:

- Daily or weekly pain intensity (for example, on a 1–10 scale)
- Flare-ups, with date, suspected triggers, and duration
- Foods eaten, focusing on new additions or eliminated items
- Additional symptoms such as digestive discomfort, fatigue, or mood changes

Many individuals notice correlations between certain foods and symptom flares, and tracking tools can clarify these links. If you find patterns, you can adjust your diet accordingly or discuss them with your healthcare provider for tailored recommendations.

Technological tools can also be helpful here. Apps designed for pain and symptom tracking, or even basic spreadsheets, can streamline the process. Over time, you might observe improvements in energy, mood, or pain that reinforce your commitment and highlight diet's role in your overall management plan.

Reviewing symptom changes with your medical team at regular intervals can further validate your efforts and provide opportunities for positive reinforcement or professional guidance if adjustments are needed.

Community Resources and Ongoing Education

Sustaining diet and lifestyle changes is considerably easier with access to community resources and educational support. Isolation can undermine motivation, while connection fosters accountability, learning, and encouragement.

Consider these avenues for community support:

1. Local or online support groups for individuals managing chronic pain or inflammatory conditions, where members share recipes, struggles, and motivation.
2. Group cooking classes with a focus on healthful, anti-inflammatory recipes.
3. Consulting a registered dietitian or nutritionist familiar with nerve pain and inflammation. Many offer group or telehealth programs.
4. Following reputable organizations or foundations providing evidence-based updates in pain management nutrition. Look for groups affiliated with neurology, rheumatology, or pain research.

Continual education is equally important. Nutrition science evolves, and staying current ensures your approach remains effective and safe. Trusted sources for ongoing learning include peer-reviewed medical journals, university-affiliated extension programs, and professional organizations.

Engaging in these communities and learning opportunities provides practical tips, emotional support, and a sense of camaraderie that makes overcoming obstacles and celebrating milestones more rewarding.

Successfully integrating an anti-inflammatory eating pattern for arachnoiditis involves more than following recipes; it's about embedding new habits into your everyday routines, adjusting as life changes, and accessing resources to stay informed and engaged. By setting realistic goals, learning to confidently handle social situations, proactively addressing challenges, systematically tracking symptoms, and tapping into educational and community networks, you can build lasting, meaningful gains for your health. Remember, persistence matters more than perfection, and every small, positive step contributes to long-term relief and improved quality of life.

Conclusion

Embracing an anti-inflammatory approach to nutrition offers important, lasting benefits for people managing arachnoiditis and chronic nerve pain. Throughout this guide, we have examined the science-backed principles behind an anti-inflammatory diet. By focusing on nutrient-dense, minimally processed foods—such as leafy greens, berries, fatty fish, and whole grains—you can help counteract inflammation, support nerve function, and promote overall well-being. A well-structured anti-inflammatory eating pattern is linked with reductions in pain severity, improved mood, and enhanced quality of life for those suffering from chronic neurological conditions.

However, lasting dietary change is rarely swift. The process of shifting eating habits takes time and patience, especially when living with a condition that may affect energy levels and daily routines. The most sustainable progress comes from gradual, consistent steps forward. Begin with manageable changes, such as introducing one new anti-inflammatory recipe per week or swapping a highly processed snack for a piece of fresh fruit. Celebrate these small victories—they add up to fundamental change over the long term.

Commitment to new dietary patterns is easier when you set specific, realistic goals. Track your meals and symptoms so you can identify what works best for you, and use setbacks as learning opportunities—not reasons to give up. Social situations, busy days, and occasional dietary lapses are inevitable, but gentle persistence will help build healthier habits over time. Remember that sustainable nutrition is a journey, not a quick fix or all-or-nothing endeavor.

As you continue to nourish your body, it remains vital to think beyond food alone. An anti-inflammatory diet is a powerful tool, but every aspect of your care deserves attention. Effective management of arachnoiditis and nerve pain typically involves a multidisciplinary approach. Collaborate with your healthcare professionals, including nutritionists, physicians, pain specialists, and physical therapists. These experts can help tailor your nutritional strategy to fit your unique needs and coordinate it with medications, movement practices, or other therapies you may require.

Ongoing communication with your care team can provide practical guidance and emotional encouragement. They can help monitor the effectiveness of your dietary changes, advise on safe supplementation, and support you as you adjust to new routines and symptom fluctuations. Integrating expert input ensures your nutritional choices remain evidence-based, adaptable, and supportive of your overall treatment goals.

Ultimately, informed nutrition is a cornerstone of sustained relief for those living with arachnoiditis and chronic nerve pain. By combining smart dietary choices with professional support, you invest in your long-term well-being. Every step, from choosing nourishing meals to reaching out for multidisciplinary care, contributes to building comfort, resilience, and renewed vitality.

FAQs

What is Arachnoiditis and how does it affect the nerves?

Arachnoiditis is a chronic pain disorder caused by inflammation of the arachnoid mater, one of the membranes protecting the brain and spinal cord. This condition most often affects nerves within the spinal canal, leading to dysfunction and ongoing neuropathic pain. Causes include spinal injury, infections, and medical procedures such as surgery or injections. Inflammation may cause nerve roots to become scarred or stick together, disrupting normal nerve signals. Symptoms include persistent burning or stabbing pain, tingling, numbness, and sometimes muscle weakness or loss of coordination. These can significantly affect daily life, with intensity fluctuating based on triggers like activity or stress. The root problem is inflammation damaging nerves, which can create a cycle of pain if not managed.

Which foods commonly worsen Arachnoiditis symptoms?

Diet can influence inflammation, which is important for those with Arachnoiditis. Foods that tend to worsen symptoms are those that promote inflammation. Refined sugars and sweetened drinks can spike blood sugar and trigger inflammatory pathways, while saturated and trans fats from fried foods and processed meats also contribute. Excess salt in processed snacks and canned foods can cause swelling and nerve irritation. Additives, preservatives, and artificial ingredients may increase sensitivity. Alcohol and high caffeine can disrupt sleep and worsen nerve pain. For those with specific intolerances like gluten or lactose, trigger foods can increase inflammation and pain. Generally, a Western diet high in processed, low-nutrient foods is linked to more pain and inflammation in nerve conditions.

How quickly can dietary changes improve nerve pain?

Improvements in nerve pain after dietary changes vary. Some people notice reduced pain or fewer flares within two to four weeks of adopting an anti-inflammatory diet, especially if they identify and eliminate specific triggers. However, for chronic or advanced cases, it may take several months of consistent effort to see significant improvements due to persistent inflammation. Tracking symptoms and consulting with healthcare professionals can help. Dietary changes are most effective alongside other treatments, such as physical therapy and medications.

Can supplements replace an anti-inflammatory diet?

Supplements can support nerve health but cannot replace a diet rich in whole, minimally processed foods. The body benefits from the vitamins, minerals, fiber, and healthy fats found in fruits, vegetables, nuts, seeds, and fish. Supplements like omega-3s, vitamin D, or magnesium may help but work best as adjuncts. Overuse of supplements without medical supervision can cause imbalances or side effects. For those with dietary restrictions, targeted supplementation may be needed, but should be guided by a healthcare provider. The foundation for nerve pain support remains a nutrient-dense, anti-inflammatory diet, with supplements reserved for specific needs.

Are nightshade vegetables safe for those with nerve pain?

Nightshades—tomatoes, potatoes, eggplants, bell peppers—contain natural compounds some believe may worsen pain in sensitive people. However, most individuals tolerate them well, and these vegetables provide valuable nutrients. There is little clinical evidence that nightshades consistently worsen nerve pain for most people with Arachnoiditis. If you suspect they contribute to your pain, try a short-term elimination and reintroduction. For most, including nightshades as part of a varied, plant-rich diet is safe unless a personal sensitivity is uncovered.

Is fasting recommended for people with Arachnoiditis?

Fasting and time-restricted eating may have anti-inflammatory effects, but recommendations for people with Arachnoiditis should be individualized. While some evidence suggests modest fasting can reduce inflammation, severe or prolonged fasting can cause unstable blood sugar and may worsen nerve symptoms. Regular, balanced meals rich in anti-inflammatory foods are generally safer. Any fasting should be discussed with a healthcare team.

Where can I find more support for dietary changes and pain management?

Support is available. Start with a registered dietitian experienced in neurological conditions. Peer support groups and national patient organizations offer resources and encouragement. Consult knowledgeable pain physicians or therapists for a holistic approach. Evidence-based health websites, books, and expert podcasts can provide further guidance. Sustainable change is easier with a supportive, multidisciplinary team and reliable resources.

References and Helpful Links

Calder, P. C.. Omega-3 fatty acids and inflammatory processes: from molecules to man. n.d.. Accessed January 27, 2026. https://eprints.soton.ac.uk/415428/

Pickering, G. et al.. Magnesium and Pain: A Review of the Literature. n.d.. Accessed January 27, 2026. https://www.mdpi.com/2072-6643/13/5/1397

Vinik, A. I. et al.. Glycemic Control and Neuropathic Pain: Clinical Implications. n.d. 20. 20. Accessed January 27, 2026. https://www.endo.theclinics.com/article/S0889-8529(13)00052-2/abstract

Callaghan, B. C. & Feldman, E. L.. Painful Diabetic Neuropathy: Current and Future Treatments. n.d.. Accessed January 27, 2026. https://www.bmj.com/content/348/bmj.g1799.abstract

Daily, J. W., Yang, M., & Park, S.. Efficacy of turmeric extracts and curcumin for alleviating the symptoms of joint arthritis: a systematic review and meta-analysis of randomized clinical trials. n.d.. Accessed January 27, 2026. https://www.liebertpub.com/doi/abs/10.1089/jmf.2016.3705

Strazzullo, P. Salt intake, stroke, and cardiovascular disease: meta-analysis of prospective studies. n.d.. Accessed January 27, 2026. https://www.bmj.com/content/339/bmj.b4567.abstract

Mayer, E. A.. Gut/brain axis and the microbiota. n.d.. Accessed January 27, 2026. https://www.jci.org/articles/view/76304

H Peng. Arachnoiditis. n.d.. Accessed January 27, 2026. https://www.ncbi.nlm.nih.gov/books/NBK555973/

What It Is, Causes, Symptoms & Treatment. n.d. 20. Accessed January 27, 2026. https://my.clevelandclinic.org/health/diseases/12062-arachnoiditis

www.ingramcontent.com/pod-product-compliance
Lightning Source LLC
LaVergne TN
LVHW022006200926
848481LV00007B/2264